The Comprehensive Air Fryer Meat Cooking Guide

Easy And Tasty Meat Air Fryer Recipes For Everyone

Ellie Sloan

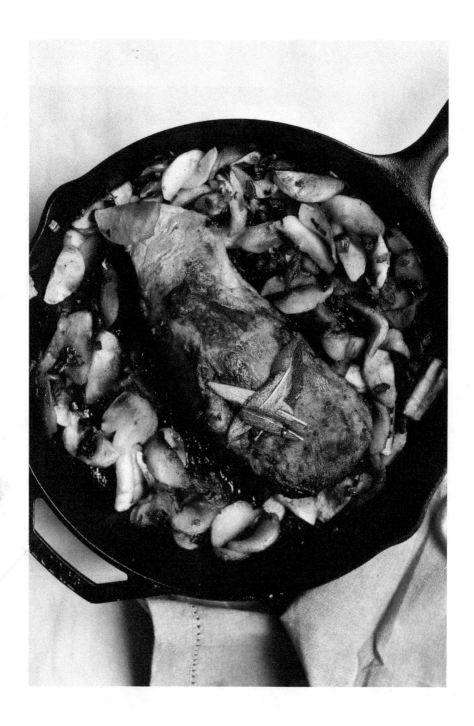

Table of contents

Ranch Chicken Thighs

Preparation Time: 10 minutes

Cooking Time: 23 minutes

Servings: 4

Ingredients:

- Chicken thighs, bone-in & skin-on
- 1/2 tbsp. ranch dressing mix

Directions:

1. Add chicken thighs into the mixing bowl and sprinkle with ranch dressing mix. Toss well to coat.
2. Spray chicken thighs with cooking spray and place into the Air Fryer basket.
3. Cook at 380°F for 23 minutes. Turn chicken halfway through.
4. Serve and enjoy.

Nutrition:

Calories 558

Fat 21.7g

Carbs 0.5g

Protein 84.6g

Taco Ranch Chicken Wings

Preparation Time: 10 minutes

Cooking Time: 30 minutes

Servings: 4

Ingredients:

- 2 lbs. chicken wings
- 1 tsp. ranch seasoning
- 1 1/2 tsp. taco seasoning
- 1 tsp. olive oil

Directions:

1. Preheat the Air Fryer to 400°F.
2. In a mixing bowl, add chicken wings, ranch seasoning, taco seasoning, and oil and toss well to coat.
3. Place chicken wings into the Air Fryer basket and cook for 15 minutes.
4. Turn chicken wings to another side and cook for 15 minutes more.

5. Serve and enjoy.

Nutrition:

Calories 444

Fat 18g

Carbs 0g

Protein 65.6g

Simple Cajun Chicken Wings

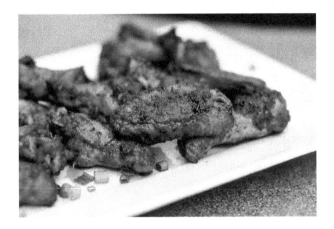

Preparation Time: 10 minutes

Cooking Time: 25 minutes

Servings: 4

Ingredients:

- 2 lbs. chicken wings
- 1/3 cup ranch dressing
- 1 tbsp. + 1/2 tsp. Cajun seasoning

Directions:

1. Rub 1 tbsp. Cajun seasoning all over chicken wings.
2. Place chicken wings into the Air Fryer basket and cook at 400°F for 25 minutes. Turn chicken wings halfway through.
3. Meanwhile, in a small bowl, mix together ranch dressing and 1 tsp. Cajun seasoning.
4. Serve chicken wings with Cajun ranch dressing.

Nutrition:

Calories 437

Fat 16.9g

Carbs 1.1g

Protein 65.9g

Simple Air Fried Chicken

Preparation Time: 10 minutes

Cooking Time: 10 minutes

Servings: 4

Ingredients:

- oz chicken, skinless and boneless
- 1/2 tsp. black pepper
- 1/2 tsp. salt
- 1/2 cup almond meal
- 1 egg, beaten

Directions:

1. Preheat the Air Fryer at 330°F.
2. Add egg in a bowl and whisk until frothy and season with pepper and salt.
3. In a shallow dish, mix together almond meal and salt.
4. Dip chicken into the egg mixture then coats with almond meal.

5. Place coated chicken into the Air Fryer basket and cook for 10 minutes.
6. Serve and enjoy.

Nutrition:

Calories 285

Fat 12.8g

Carbs 3.7g

Protein 38.1g

Buffalo Wings

Preparation Time: **5 minutes**

Cooking Time: **15 minutes**

Servings: **4**

Ingredients:

- 32 oz chicken wings
- 1/4 cup hot sauce
- tbsp. grass-fed butter, melted
- Salt

Directions:

1. Add chicken wings into the bowl. Pour hot sauce and butter over chicken wings and toss well.
2. Place marinated chicken wings into the refrigerator for 1-2 hours.
3. Preheat the Air Fryer at 400°F for 3 minutes
4. Place marinated chicken wings into the Air Fryer basket and cook for 12 minutes. shake basket halfway through.
5. Serve and enjoy.

Nutrition:

Calories 678

Fat 34 g

Carbs 0.4 g

Protein 87.7 g

Honey Lime Chicken Wings

Preparation Time: 10 minutes

Cooking Time: 50 minutes

Servings: 6

Ingredients:

- 2 lbs chicken wings
- tbsp. fresh lime juice
- salt and black pepper
- 1/4 tsp. white pepper powder
- tbsp. honey

Directions:

1. In a bowl, place all the ingredients and coat well.
2. Place marinated chicken wings into the refrigerator for 1-2 hours.
3. Preheat the Air Fryer to 360°F.

4. Place marinated chicken wings into the Air Fryer basket and cook for 12 minutes. Shake Air Fryer basket halfway through.

5. Turn temperature to 400°F and cook for 3 minutes more. Serve and enjoy.

Nutrition:

Calories 311

Fat 11.2g

Carbs 6.1g

Protein 43.8g

Simple Chicken Drumsticks

Preparation Time: 10 minutes

Cooking Time: 16 minutes

Servings: 4

Ingredients:

- 1 1/2 lbs chicken drumsticks
- tbsp. chicken seasoning
- 1 tsp. black pepper
- 1 tbsp. olive oil
- 1 tsp. salt

Directions:

1. In a small bowl, mix together chicken seasoning, olive oil, pepper, and salt.
2. Rub seasoning mixture all over the chicken.
3. Place seasoned chicken into the Air Fryer basket and cook for 10 minutes. Flip halfway through.

4. Turn temperature to 300°F and cook for 6 minutes more. Serve and enjoy.

Nutrition:

Calories 319

Fat 13.2g

Carbs 0.3g

Protein 46.8g

Healthy Chicken Wings

Preparation Time: 10 minutes

Cooking Time: 25 minutes

Servings: 4

Ingredients:

- lbs. chicken wings
- 1 tbsp. pepper
- 1 tbsp. garlic powder
- tbsp. seasoning salt

Directions:

1. In a bowl, mix all of the ingredients except for the chicken wings.
2. Add chicken wings in a bowl and toss until well coated.
3. Preheat the Air Fryer at 370°F for 5 minutes.
4. Put the chicken wings into the basket of the Air Fryer and cook for 20 minutes. Shake basket halfway through.
5. Serve and enjoy.

Nutrition:

Calories 442

Fat 16.9g

Carbs 2.6g

Protein 66.1g

Thai Chicken Thighs

Preparation Time: 10 minutes

Cooking Time: 20 minutes

Servings: 4

Ingredients:

- 1 lb. chicken thighs, boneless and skinless
- tsp. ginger, minced
- garlic cloves, chopped
- 1/2 cup coconut milk
- tbsp. curry paste

Directions:

1. Add all ingredients into the zip-lock bag and shake well and place bag in the refrigerator for overnight.
2. Add marinated chicken and the sauce in a pie dish.
3. Place dish in Air Fryer and cook for 20 minutes at 165°F. Serve and enjoy.

Nutrition:

Calories 341

Fat 20g

Carbs 5.2g

Protein 34.1g

Chicken Patties

Preparation Time: 10 minutes

Cooking Time: 13 minutes

Servings: 8

Ingredients:

- lbs ground chicken
- 1 cup homemade salsa
- 1/2 small onion, chopped
- 1 1/2 cups egg whites
- Salt and Pepper

Directions:

1. Add egg whites, salsa, and onion into the blender and blend until combined.
2. Add ground chicken and egg mixture into the large mixing bowl. Season with pepper and salt and mix until well combined.
3. Make small patties from meat mixture.

4. Spray Air Fryer basket with cooking spray.

5. Place chicken patties in Air Fryer and cook for 12-13 minutes at 345°F. Cook in batches. Serve and enjoy.

Nutrition:

Calories 357

Fat 12.7g

Carbs 2.8g

Protein 54.7g

Cajun Seasoned Chicken Drumsticks

Preparation Time: 5 minutes

Cooking Time: 15 minutes

Servings: 2

Ingredients:

- chicken drumsticks, skinless
- 1 tbsp. Cajun seasoning
- tsp. olive oil

Directions:

1. Add all ingredients to the zip-lock bag. Shake bag well and place in refrigerator for half hour.
2. Place marinated chicken drumsticks in Air Fryer basket and cook for 15 minutes at 400°F.
3. Serve and enjoy.

Nutrition:

Calories 118

Fat 7.3g

Carbs 0g

Protein 12.7g

Honey Garlic Chicken

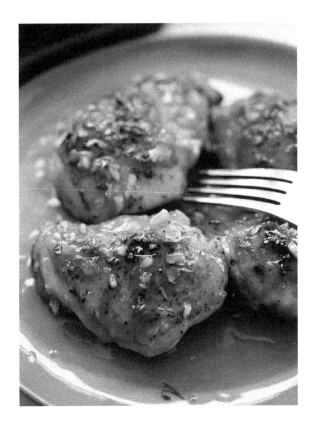

Preparation Time: 10 minutes

Cooking Time: 15 minutes

Servings: 2

Ingredients:

- Chicken drumsticks, skinless
- 1/2 tsp. garlic, minced
- tsp. honey
- tsp. olive oil

Directions:

1. Put all of the ingredients to a bowl and mix until well coated.
2. Place chicken in refrigerator for half hour.
3. Place marinated chicken into the Air Fryer and cook for 15 minutes at 400°F.
4. Serve and enjoy.

Nutrition:

Calories 140

Fat 7.3g

Carbs 6g

Protein 12.7g

Sriracha Chicken Wings

Preparation Time: 10 minutes

Cooking Time: 35 minutes

Servings: 2

Ingredients:

- 1 lb. chicken wings
- 1/2 lime juice
- 1 tbsp. grass-fed butter
- tbsp. sriracha sauce
- 1/4 cup honey

Directions:

1. Preheat the Air Fryer to 360°F.
2. Add chicken wings in Air Fryer basket and cook for 30 minutes.
3. Meanwhile, in a pan, add all remaining ingredients and bring to boil for 3 minutes.

4. Once chicken wings are done then toss with sauce and serve.

Nutrition:

Calories 711

Fat 32.6g

Carbs 35.9g

Protein 65.8g

Sweet & Spicy Chicken Wings

Preparation Time: 10 minutes

Cooking Time: 20 minutes

Servings: 8

Ingredients:

- lbs. chicken wings
- tbsp. honey
- 1/2 cup buffalo sauce
- tbsp. grass-fed butter, melted
- Salt and Pepper

Directions:

1. Put the chicken wings into the basket of the Air Fryer and cook for 20 minutes at 400°F. Shake Air Fryer basket 2 times during the cooking.
2. In a large bowl, combine together honey, buffalo sauce, butter, pepper, and salt.

3. Add cooked chicken wings into the bowl and toss until well coated with sauce.
4. Serve and enjoy.

Nutrition:

Calories 262

Fat 11.7g

Carbs 4.6g

Protein 32.9g

Ginger Garlic Chicken

Preparation Time: 10 minutes

Cooking Time: 30 minutes

Servings: 2

Ingredients:

- chicken thighs, skinless and boneless
- 1/2 tsp. ground ginger
- 1 garlic clove, minced
- tbsp. ketchup
- 1/2 cup honey

Directions:

1. Cut chicken thighs into the small pieces and place them into the Air Fryer basket and cook for 25 minutes at 390°F.
2. Meanwhile, in a pan heat together honey, ketchup, garlic, and ground ginger for 4-5 minutes.
3. Once the chicken is cooked then transfer into the mixing bowl.

4. Pour honey mixture over the chicken and toss until well coated.
5. Serve and enjoy.

Nutrition:

Calories 554

Fat 16.3g

Carbs 37.2g

Protein 63.7g

Salt and Pepper Wings

Preparation Time: 5 minutes

Cooking Time: 10 minutes

Servings: 4

Ingredients:

- 2 tsp.s salt
- 2 tsp.s fresh ground pepper
- 2 lb. chicken wings

Directions:

1. In a bowl, mix the salt and pepper.
2. Add the wings to the bowl and mix with your hands to coat every last one.
3. Put 8 to 10 wings in the Air Fryer basket that has been sprayed with nonstick cooking spray. Set for 350°F (there is no need to preheat) and cook about 15 minutes, turning once at 7 minutes.
4. Repeat with rest of wings and serve hot.

Nutrition:

Calories 342

Fat 14.8g

Carbs 1g

Protein 49.2g

Parmesan Chicken Wings

Preparation Time: 10 minutes

Cooking Time: 25 minutes

Servings: 4

Ingredients:

- 1 1/2 lbs. chicken wings
- 3/4 tbsp. garlic powder
- 1/4 cup parmesan cheese, grated
- 2 tbsp. arrowroot powder
- Salt and Pepper

Directions:

1. Preheat the Air Fryer to 380°F.
2. In a bowl, mix the garlic powder, parmesan cheese, arrowroot powder, pepper, and salt together. Add chicken wings and toss until well coated.
3. Put the chicken wings into the Air Fryer basket. Spray top of chicken wings with cooking spray.

4. Select chicken and press start. Shake Air Fryer basket halfway through. Serve and enjoy.

Nutrition:

Calories 38

Fat 15.3g

Carbs 5.6g

Protein 53.5g

Western Chicken Wings

Preparation Time: 10 minutes

Cooking Time: 15 minutes

Servings: 4

Ingredients:

- 2 lbs. chicken wings
- 1 tsp. Herb de Provence
- 1 tsp. paprika
- 1/2 cup parmesan cheese, grated
- Salt and Pepper

Directions:

1. Add cheese, paprika, herb de Provence, pepper, and salt into the large mixing bowl. Place the chicken wings into the bowl and toss well to coat.
2. Preheat the Air Fryer to 350°F.
3. Place the chicken wings into the Air Fryer basket. Spray top of chicken wings with cooking spray.

4. Cook chicken wings for 15 minutes. Turn chicken wings halfway through. Serve and enjoy.

Nutrition:

Calories 473

Fat 19.6g

Carbs 0.8g

Protein 69.7g

Perfect Chicken Thighs Dinner

Preparation Time: 10 minutes

Cooking Time: 15 minutes

Servings: 4

Ingredients:

- 4 chicken thighs, bone-in & skinless
- 1/4 tsp. ground ginger
- 2 tsp. paprika
- 2 tsp. garlic powder
- salt and pepper

Directions:

1. Preheat the Air Fryer to 400°F.
2. In a bowl, mix ginger, paprika, garlic powder, pepper, and salt together and rub all over chicken thighs.
3. Spray chicken thighs with cooking spray.
4. Place chicken thighs into the Air Fryer basket and cook for 10 minutes.

5. Turn chicken thighs and cook for 5 minutes more. Serve and enjoy.

Nutrition:

Calories 286

Fat 11g

Carbs 1.8g

Protein 42.7g

Perfectly Spiced Chicken Tenders

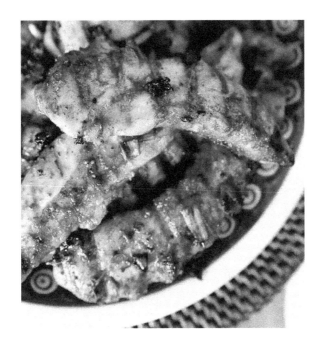

Preparation Time: 10 minutes

Cooking Time: 13 minutes

Servings: 4

Ingredients:

- 6 chicken tenders

45

- 1 tsp. onion powder
- 1 tsp. garlic powder
- 1 tsp. paprika
- 1 tsp. kosher salt

Directions:

1. Preheat the Air Fryer to 380°F.
2. In a bowl, mix onion powder, garlic powder, paprika, and salt together and rub all over chicken tenders.
3. Spray chicken tenders with cooking spray.
4. Place chicken tenders into the Air Fryer basket and cook for 13 minutes. Serve and enjoy.

Nutrition:

Calories 423

Fat 16.4g

Carbs 1.5g

Protein 63.7g

Flavorful Steak

Preparation Time: 10 minutes

Cooking Time: 18 minutes

Servings: 2

Ingredients:

- 2 steaks, rinsed and pat dry
- ½ tsp. garlic powder
- 1 tsp. olive oil
- Pepper
- Salt

Directions:

1. Brush steaks with olive oil and season with garlic powder, pepper, and salt.
2. Preheat the Air Fryer oven to 400°F.
3. Place steaks on Air Fryer oven pan and air fry for 10-18 minutes. Turn halfway through. Serve and enjoy.

Nutrition:

Calories	361
Fat	10.9g
Carbs	0.5g

Protein 61.6g

Easy Rosemary Lamb Chops

Preparation Time: 10 minutes

Cooking Time: 6 minutes

Servings: 4

Ingredients:

- 4 lamb chops
- 2 tbsp. dried rosemary
- ¼ cup fresh lemon juice
- Pepper
- Salt

Directions:

1. In a small bowl, mix together lemon juice, rosemary, pepper, and salt.
2. Brush lemon juice rosemary mixture over lamb chops.
3. Place lamb chops on Air Fryer oven tray and air fry at 400°F for 3 minutes.

4. Turn lamb chops to the other side and cook for 3 minutes more. Serve and enjoy.

Nutrition:

Calories 267

Fat 21.7g

Carbs 1.4g

Protein 16.9g

BBQ Pork Ribs

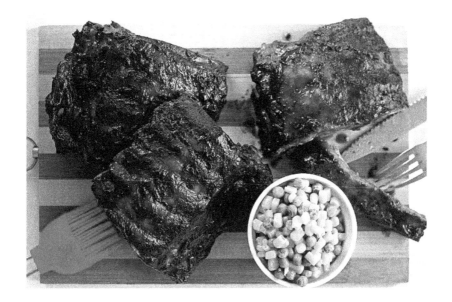

Preparation Time: 10 minutes

Cooking Time: 12 minutes

Servings: 6

Ingredients:

- 1 slab baby back pork ribs, cut into pieces
- ½ cup BBQ sauce

- ½ tsp. paprika
- Salt

Directions:

1. Add pork ribs in a mixing bowl.
2. Add BBQ sauce, paprika, and salt over pork ribs and coat well and set aside for 30 minutes.
3. Preheat the Air Fryer oven to 350°F.
4. Arrange marinated pork ribs on Air Fryer oven pan and cook for 10-12 minutes. Turn halfway through. Serve and enjoy.

Nutrition:

Calories 145

Fat 7g

Carbs 10g

Protein 9g

Juicy Steak Bites

Preparation Time: 10 minutes

Cooking Time: 9 minutes

Servings: 4

Ingredients:

- 1 lb. sirloin steak, sliced into bite-size pieces
- 1 tbsp. steak seasoning
- 1 tbsp. olive oil
- Pepper
- Salt

Directions:

1. Preheat the instant Air Fryer oven to 390°F.
2. Add steak pieces into the large mixing bowl. Add steak seasoning, oil, pepper, and salt over steak pieces and toss until well coated.
3. Transfer steak pieces on Air Fryer pan and air fry for 5 minutes.

4. Turn steak pieces to the other side and cook for 4 minutes more. Serve and enjoy.

Nutrition:

Calories 241

Fat 10.6g

Carbs 0g

Protein 34.4g

Greek Lamb Chops

Preparation Time: 10 minutes

Cooking Time: 10 minutes

Servings: 4

Ingredients:

- 2 lbs. lamb chops
- 2 tsp. garlic, minced
- 1 ½ tsp. dried oregano
- ¼ cup fresh lemon juice
- salt and pepper

Directions:

1. Add lamb chops in a mixing bowl. Add remaining ingredients over the lamb chops and coat well.
2. Arrange lamb chops on the Air Fryer oven tray and cook at 400°F for 5 minutes.
3. Turn lamb chops and cook for 5 minutes more. Serve and enjoy.

Nutrition:

Calories	538
Fat	29.4g
Carbs	1.3g
Protein 64g	

Easy Beef Roast

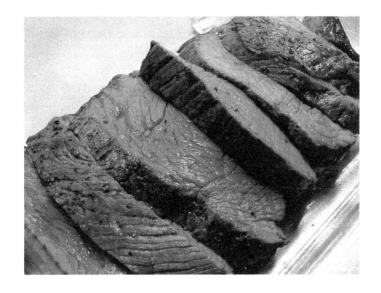

Preparation Time: 10 minutes

Cooking Time: 45 minutes

Servings: 6

Ingredients:

- 2 ½ lbs. beef roast
- 2 tbsp. Italian seasoning

Directions:

1. Arrange roast on the rotisserie spite.
2. Rub roast with Italian seasoning then insert into the Air Fryer oven.
3. Air fry at 350°F for 45 minutes or until the internal temperature of the roast reaches to 145°F. Slice and serve.

Nutrition:

Calories 365

Fat 13.2g

Carbs 0.5g

Protein 57.4g

Beef Jerky

Preparation Time: 10 minutes

Cooking Time: 4 hours

Servings: 4

Ingredients:

- 2 lbs. London broil, sliced thinly
- 1 tsp. onion powder
- 3 tbsp. brown sugar
- 3 tbsp. soy sauce
- 1 tsp. olive oil

Directions:

1. Add all ingredients except meat in the large zip-lock bag.
2. Mix until well combined. Add meat in the bag.
3. Seal bag and massage gently to cover the meat with marinade.
4. Let marinate the meat for 1 hour.

5. Arrange marinated meat slices on Air Fryer tray and dehydrate at 160°F for 4 hours.

Nutrition:

Calories 133

Fat 4.7g

Carbs 9.4g

Protein 13.4g

Simple Beef Patties

Preparation Time: 10 minutes

Cooking Time: 13 minutes

Servings: 4

Ingredients:

- 1 lb. ground beef
- ½ tsp. garlic powder
- ¼ tsp. onion powder
- Salt and Pepper

Directions:

1. Preheat the Air Fryer oven to 400°F.
2. Add ground meat, garlic powder, onion powder, pepper, and salt into the mixing bowl and mix until well combined.
3. Make even shape patties from meat mixture and arrange on Air Fryer pan.

4. Place pan in Air Fryer oven. Cook patties for 10 minutes. Turn patties after 5 minutes. Serve and enjoy.

Nutrition:

Calories 212

Fat 7.1g

Carbs 0.4g

Protein 34.5g

Panko-Breaded Pork Chops

Preparation Time: 5 minutes

Cooking Time: 12 minutes

Servings: 6

Ingredients:

- 5 (3½- to 5 oz.) pork chops (bone-in or boneless)
- salt and pepper
- ¼ cup all-purpose flour
- 2 tbsp. panko bread crumbs
- Cooking oil

Directions:

1. Season the pork chops with salt and pepper to taste.
2. Sprinkle the flour on both sides of the pork chops, then coat both sides with panko bread crumbs.
3. Put the pork chops in the Air Fryer. Stacking them is okay.

4. Spray the pork chops with cooking oil. Cook for 6 minutes at 365°F.
5. Halfway through, flip the pork chops. Cook for an additional 6 minutes
6. Cool before serving.
7. Typically, bone-in pork chops are juicier than boneless. If you prefer really juicy pork chops, use bone-in.

Nutrition:

Calories 246

Fat 13g

Carbs 11g

Protein 26g

Crispy Roast Garlic-Salt Pork

Preparation Time: 5 minutes

Cooking Time: 45 minutes

Servings: 4

Ingredients:

- 1 tsp. Chinese five spice powder
- 1 tsp. white pepper
- 2 lb. pork belly
- 2 tsp.s garlic salt

Directions:

1. Preheat the Air Fryer to 390°F.
2. Mix all of the seasonings in a bowl to create the dry rub.
3. Score the skin of the pork belly with a knife and season the entire pork with the spice rub.
4. Place in the Air Fryer basket and cook for 40 to 45 minutes until the skin is crispy. Chop before serving.

Nutrition:

Calories 785

Fat 80.7g

Carbs 7g

Protein 14.2g

Beef Rolls

Preparation Time: 10 minutes

Cooking Time: 14 minutes

Servings: 4

Ingredients:

- 2 lb. beef steak, opened and flattened with a meat tenderizer
- Salt and black pepper to the taste
- 3 oz. red bell pepper, roasted and chopped
- 6 slices provolone cheese
- 3 tbsp. pesto

Directions:

1. Arrange flattened beef steak on a cutting board, spread pesto all over, add cheese in a single layer, add bell peppers, salt and pepper to the taste.
2. Roll your steak, secure with toothpicks, season again with salt and pepper, place roll in your Air Fryer's

basket and cook at 400°F for 14 minutes, rotating roll halfway.

3. Leave aside to cool down, cut into 2-inch smaller rolls, arrange on a platter and serve them as an appetizer. Enjoy!

Nutrition:

Calories 23

Fat 17g

Carbs 12g

Protein 10g

Homemade Corned Beef with Onions

Preparation Time: 5 minutes

Cooking Time: 50 minutes

Servings: 4

Ingredients:

- Salt and pepper to taste
- 1 cup water
- 1-lb. corned beef brisket, cut into chunks
- 1 tbsp. Dijon mustard
- 1 small onion, chopped

Directions:

1. Preheat the Air Fryer to 400°F.
2. Place all ingredients in a baking dish that will fit in the Air Fryer.
3. Cover with foil. Cook for 35 minutes.
4. Remove foil, mix well, turnover beef, and continue cooking for another 15 minutes.

Nutrition:

Calories 238

Carbs 3.1g

Protein 17.2g

Fat 17.1g

Crisp Ribs

Preparation Time: 10 minutes

Cooking Time: 50 minutes

Serving: 2

Ingredients:

- 1 rack of pork ribs

Rub:

- 1 1/2 cup broth
- 3 tbsp. Liquid Smoke
- 1 cup Barbecue Sauce

Directions:

1. Rub the rib rack with spice rub generously.
2. Pour the liquid into the Air Fryer. Set an Air Fryer Basket into the Pot and place the rib rack in the basket.

3. Put on the pressure-cooking lid (if available) and seal it.
4. Hit the "Pressure Button" and select 30 minutes of Cooking Time, then press "Start."
5. Once the Air Fryer, do a quick release and remove its lid.
6. Remove the ribs and rub them with barbecue sauce. Empty the pot and place the Air Fryer Basket in it.
7. Set the ribs in the basket, and Air fry them at 370°F for 20 minutes. Serve.

Nutrition:

Calories 306

Fat 6.4g

Carbs 46g

Protein 14.7g

Roast Beef

Preparation Time: 10 minutes

Cooking Time: 15 minutes

Serving: 4

Ingredients:

- 2 lb. beef roast top
- oil for spraying
- Rub
- Salt and pepper to taste
- 2 tsp. garlic powder
- 1 tsp. summer savory

Directions:

1. Whisk all the rub ingredients: in a small bowl.
2. Liberally rub this mixture over the roast.
3. Place an Air Fryer Basket in the Air Fryer and layer it with cooking oil.

4. Set the seasoned roast in the Air Fryer Basket. Put on the Air Fryer lid and seal it.

5. Hit the "Air fry Button" and select 20 minutes of Cooking Time at 370°F, then press "Start."

6. Once the Air Fryer beeps, remove its lid. Turn the roast and continue Air Fryer for another 15 minutes. Serve warm.

Nutrition:

Calories 427

Fat 14.2g

Carbs 1.4g

Protein 69.1g

Basic Pork Chops

Preparation Time: 10 minutes

Cooking Time: 15 minutes

Serving: 4

Ingredients:

- 4 pork chops, bone-in
- 1 tbsp. olive oil
- 1 tsp. kosher salt
- 1/2 tsp. black pepper

Directions:

1. Liberally season the pork chops with olive oil, salt, and black pepper.
2. Place the pork chops in the basket and spray them with cooking spray.
3. Set the Air Fryer Basket in the Air Fryer. Put on the Air Fryer lid and seal it.

4. Hit the "Air fry Button" and select 15 minutes of Cooking Time at 360°F, then press "Start."
5. Once the Air Fryer beeps, remove its lid, serve and enjoy.

Nutrition:

Calories 28

Fat 23.4g

Carbs 0.2g

Protein 18g

Breaded Pork Chops

Preparation Time: 10 minutes

Cooking Time: 18 minutes

Serving: 4

Ingredients:

- 4 boneless, center-cut pork chops, 1-inch thick
- 1 tsp. Cajun seasoning
- 1 1/2 cups garlic-flavored croutons
- 2 eggs
- cooking spray

Directions:

1. Grind croutons in a food processor until it forms crumbs.
2. Season the pork chops with Cajun seasoning liberally.
3. Beat eggs in a shallow tray then dip the pork chops in the egg.
4. Coat the dipped chops in the crouton crumbs.

5. Place the breaded pork chops in the basket of the Air Fryer.
6. Set the Air Fryer Basket and spray the chops with cooking oil.
7. Put on the Air Fryer lid and seal it.
8. Hit the "Air fry Button" and select 18 minutes of Cooking Time at 370°F.
9. Once the Air Fryer beeps, remove its lid and serve.

Nutrition:

Calories 301

Fat 12.4g

Carbs 12.2g

Protein 32.2g

Beef and Balsamic Marinade

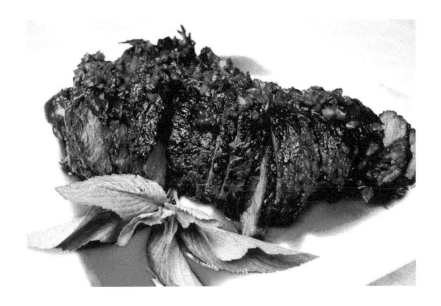

Preparation Time: 5 minutes

Cooking Time: 40 minutes

Servings: 4

Ingredients:

- 4 medium beef steaks
- 3 garlic cloves; minced

- 1 cup balsamic vinegar
- 2 tbsp. olive oil
- Salt and black pepper to taste.

Directions:

1. Take a bowl and mix steaks with the rest of the ingredients and toss.
2. Transfer the steaks to your Air Fryer's basket and cook at 390°F for 35 minutes, flipping them halfway
3. Divide among plates and serve with a side salad.

Nutrition:

Calories 273

Fat 14g

Carbs 6g

Protein 19g

Crispy Brats

Preparation Time: 5 minutes

Cooking Time: 15 minutes

Servings: 4

Ingredients:

- 4 x 3-oz. beef bratwursts

Directions:

1. Place brats into the Air Fryer basket.
2. Adjust the temperature to 375°F and set the timer for 15 minutes.

Nutrition:

Calories 286

Fat 28g

Protein 18g

Carbs 0g

Basil Pork Chops

Preparation Time: 5 minutes

Cooking Time: 30 minutes

Servings: 4

Ingredients:

- 4 pork chops
- 2 tsp. basil; dried
- ½ tsp. chili powder
- 2 tbsp. olive oil
- A pinch of salt and black pepper

Directions:

1. In a pan that fits your Air Fryer, mix all the ingredients, toss.
2. Introduce in the fryer and cook at 400°F for 25 minutes. Divide everything between plates and serve

Nutrition:

Calories 27

Fat 13g

Carbs 6g

Protein 18g

Beef and Radishes

Preparation Time: 5 minutes

Cooking Time: 15 minutes

Servings: 2

Ingredients:

- 1 lb. radishes, quartered
- 2 cups corned beef, cooked and shredded
- 2 spring onions; chopped
- 2 garlic cloves; minced
- A pinch of salt and black pepper

Directions:

1. In a pan that fits your Air Fryer, mix the beef with the rest of the ingredients, toss.
2. Put the pan in the fryer and cook at 390°F for 15 minutes
3. Divide everything into bowls and serve.

Nutrition:

Calories 267

Fat 13g

Carbs 5g

Protein 15g

Herbed Pork Chops

Preparation Time: 5 minutes

Cooking Time: 25 minutes

Servings: 4

Ingredients:

- 4 pork chops
- 2 tsp. basil; dried
- ½ tsp. chili powder
- 2 tbsp. olive oil
- A pinch of salt and black pepper

Directions:

1. In a pan that fits your Air Fryer, mix all the ingredients, toss.
2. Introduce in the fryer and cook at 400°F for 25 minutes. Divide everything between plates and serve

Nutrition:

Calories 274

Fat 13g

Carbs 6g

Protein 18g

Beef Tenderloin

Preparation Time: 5 minutes

Cooking Time: 30 minutes

Servings: 6

Ingredients:

- 1 (2-lb. beef tenderloin, trimmed of visible fat
- 2 tbsp. salted butter; melted.
- 2 tsp. minced roasted garlic
- 3 tbsp. ground 4-peppercorn blend

Directions:

1. In a small bowl, mix the butter and roasted garlic. Brush it over the beef tenderloin.
2. Place the ground peppercorns onto a plate and roll the tenderloin through them, creating a crust. Place tenderloin into the Air Fryer basket

3. Adjust the temperature to 400°F and set the timer for 25 minutes. Flip the tenderloin halfway through cooking. Set aside for 10 minutes before slicing.

Nutrition:

Calories	289
Fat	18g
Protein	37g
Carbs 5g	

Honey Mustard Pork Tenderloin

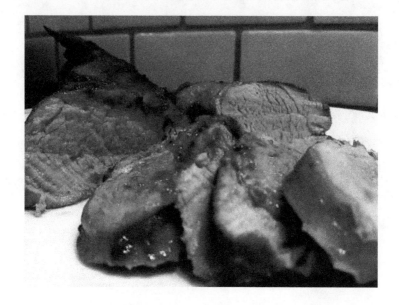

Preparation Time: 15 minutes

Cooking Time: 25 minutes

Servings: 3

Ingredients:

- 1-lb. pork tenderloin
- 1 tbsp. garlic, minced

- 2 tbsp. soy sauce
- 2 tbsp. honey
- 1 tbsp. Dijon mustard
- 1 tbsp. grain mustard
- 1 tsp. Sriracha sauce

Directions:

1. In a large bowl, add all the ingredients except pork and mix well.
2. Add the pork tenderloin and coat with the mixture generously.
3. Refrigerate to marinate for 2-3 hours.
4. Remove the pork tenderloin from bowl, reserving the marinade.
5. Place the pork tenderloin onto the lightly greased cooking tray.
6. Arrange the drip pan in the bottom of the Air Fryer Oven cooking chamber.
7. Air fry for 25 minutes at 380°F.
8. Every few minutes, turn the pork and oat with the reserved marinade.
9. When cooking time is complete, remove the tray from Air Fryer and place the pork tenderloin onto a platter for about 10 minutes before slicing.

10. With a sharp knife, cut the pork tenderloin into desired sized slices and serve.

Nutrition:

Calories 277

Fat 5.7g

Carbs 14.2g

Protein 40.7g

Seasoned Pork Chops

Preparation Time: 10 minutes

Cooking Time: 12 minutes

Servings: 4

Ingredients:

- 4 (6 oz.) boneless pork chops
- 2 tbsp. pork rub
- 1 tbsp. olive oil

Directions:

1. Coat both sides of the pork chops with the oil and then, rub with the pork rub.
2. Place the pork chops onto the lightly greased cooking tray.
3. Arrange the drip pan in the bottom of the Air Fryer Oven cooking chamber.
4. Air fry for 12 minutes at 400°F.
5. After 4-5 minutes, turn the pork chops.

6. When cooking time is complete, remove the tray from Air Fryer and serve hot.

Nutrition:

Calories 285

Fat 9.5g

Carbs 1.5g

Protein 44.5g

Crusted Rack of Lamb

Preparation Time: 15 minutes

Cooking Time: 19 minutes

Servings: 4

Ingredients:

- 1 rack of lamb, trimmed all fat and frenched
- Salt and ground black pepper, as required
- 1/3 cup pistachios, chopped finely
- 2 tbsp. panko breadcrumbs
- 2 tsp.s fresh thyme, chopped finely
- 1 tsp. fresh rosemary, chopped finely
- 1 tbsp. butter, melted
- 1 tbsp. Dijon mustard

Directions:

1. Insert the rotisserie rod through the rack on the meaty side of the ribs, right next to the bone.

2. Insert the rotisserie forks, one on each side of the rod to secure the rack.

3. Season the rack with salt and black pepper evenly.

4. Arrange the drip pan in the bottom of the Air Fryer Oven cooking chamber.

5. Set the timer for 12 minutes at 380°F.

6. When the display shows "Add Food" press the red lever down and load the left side of the rod into the Air Fryer.

7. Now, slide the rod's left side into the groove along the metal bar so it doesn't move. Then, close the door and touch "Rotate".

8. Meanwhile, in a small bowl, mix together the remaining ingredients except the mustard.

9. When cooking time is complete, remove the rack from Air Fryer and brush the meaty side with the mustard.

10. Then, coat the pistachio mixture on all sides of the rack and press firmly.

11. Now, place the rack of lamb onto the cooking tray, meat side up.

12. Air fry for 7 minutes at 380°F.

13. When cooking time is complete, remove the tray from Air Fryer and place the rack onto a cutting board for at least 10 minutes.

14. Cut the rack into individual chops and serve.

Nutrition:

Calories 824

Fat 39.3g

Carbs 10.3g

Protein 72g

Lamb Burgers

Preparation Time: 15 minutes

Cooking Time: 8 minutes

Servings: 6

Ingredients:

- 2 lb. ground lamb
- 1 tbsp. onion powder
- Salt and ground black pepper, as required

Directions:

1. In a bowl, add all the ingredients and mix well.
2. Make 6 equal-sized patties from the mixture.
3. Arrange the patties onto a cooking tray.
4. Arrange the drip pan in the bottom of the Air Fryer Oven cooking chamber.
5. Air fry for 8 minutes at 360°F.
6. After 4 minutes, turn the burgers.

7. When cooking time is complete, remove the tray from Air Fryer and serve hot.

Nutrition:

Calories	285
Fat	11.1g
Carbs	0.9g

Protein 42.6g

Pork Taquitos

Preparation Time: 10 minutes

Cooking Time: 16 minutes

Servings: 8

Ingredients:

- 1 juiced lime
- 10 whole wheat tortillas
- 2 ½ C. shredded mozzarella cheese
- 30 oz. of cooked and shredded pork tenderloin

Directions:

1. Ensure your Air Fryer is preheated to 380°F.
2. Drizzle pork with lime juice and gently mix.
3. Heat up tortillas in the microwave with a dampened paper towel to soften.
4. Add about 3 oz. of pork and ¼ cup of shredded cheese to each tortilla. Tightly roll them up. Spray the Air Fryer basket with a bit of olive oil.

5. Set temperature to 380°F, and set time to 10 minutes. Air fry taquitos 7-10 minutes till tortillas turn a slight golden color, making sure to flip halfway through cooking process.

Nutrition:

Calories 309

Fat 11g

Protein 21g

Sugar 2g

Cajun Bacon Pork Loin Fillet

Preparation Time: 10 minutes

Cooking Time: 20 minutes

Servings: 6

Ingredients:

- 1½ lb. pork loin fillet or pork tenderloin
- 3 tbsp. olive oil
- 2 tbsp. Cajun Spice Mix
- Salt
- 6 slices bacon
- Olive oil spray

Directions:

1. Cut the pork in half so that it will fit in the Air Fryer basket.
2. Place both pieces of meat in a resealable plastic bag. Add the oil, Cajun seasoning, and salt to taste, if using. Seal the bag and massage to coat all of the

meat with the oil and seasonings. Marinate in the refrigerator for at least 1 hour or up to 24 hours.

3. Remove the pork from the bag and wrap 3 bacon slices around each piece. Spray the Air Fryer basket with olive oil spray. Place the meat in the Air Fryer. Set the Air Fryer to 350°F for 15 minutes. Increase the temperature to 400°F for 5 minutes. Use a meat thermometer to ensure the meat has reached an internal temperature of 145°F.

4. Let the meat rest for 10 minutes. Slice into 6 medallions and serve.

Nutrition:

Calories 355 kcal

Fat 22.88g

Protein 34.83g

Carbs 0.6g

Porchetta-Style Pork Chops

Preparation Time: 10 minutes

Cooking Time: 15 minutes

Servings: 2

Ingredients:

- 1 tbsp. extra-virgin olive oil
- Grated zest of 1 lemon
- 2 cloves garlic, minced
- 2 tsp.s chopped fresh rosemary
- 1 tsp. finely chopped fresh sage
- 1 tsp. fennel seeds, lightly crushed
- ¼ to ½ tsp. red pepper flakes
- 1 tsp. kosher salt
- 1 tsp. black pepper
- (8 oz.) center-cut bone-in pork chops, about 1 inch thick

Directions:

1. In a small bowl, combine the olive oil, zest, garlic, rosemary, sage, fennel seeds, red pepper, salt, and

black pepper. Stir, crushing the herbs with the back of a spoon, until a paste forms. Spread the seasoning mix on both sides of the pork chops.

2. Place the chops in the Air Fryer basket. Set the Air Fryer to 375°F for 15 minutes. Use a meat thermometer to ensure the chops have reached an internal temperature of 145°F.

Nutrition:

Calories 200

Fat 9.69g

Protein 23.45g

Carbs 4.46g

Apricot Glazed Pork Tenderloins

Preparation Time: 5 minutes

Cooking Time: 30 minutes

Servings: 3

Ingredients:

- 1 tsp. salt
- 1/2 tsp. pepper
- 1 lb. pork tenderloin
- 2 tbsp. minced fresh rosemary or 1 tbsp. dried rosemary, crushed
- 2 tbsp. olive oil, divided
- 1 garlic cloves, minced
- Apricot Glaze Ingredients
- 1 cup apricot preserves
- 3 garlic cloves, minced
- 4 tbsp. lemon juice

Directions:

1. Mix well pepper, salt, garlic, oil, and rosemary. Brush all over pork. If needed cut pork crosswise in half to fit in Air Fryer. Lightly grease baking pan of Air Fryer with cooking spray. Add pork.
2. For 3 minutes per side, brown pork in a preheated 390°F Air Fryer. Meanwhile, mix well all glaze Ingredients in a small bowl. Baste pork every 5 minutes. Cook for 20 minutes at 330°F. Serve and enjoy.

Nutrition:

Calories 45

Protein 43.76g

Fat 16.71g

Carbs 33.68g